Contents

What Is Acupuncture?

For more than 5,000 years, acupuncturists have treated many diseases or dysfunctions of the body by inserting fine needles into the skin at specific points. The needles stimulate these acupuncture points to normalize physiological functions, to modify or prevent the perception of pain, and to encourage the body's own healing abilities. The classic theory supporting Traditional Chinese Medicine uses a holistic approach to treat the patient. The life force which circulates throughout the body is made up of qi (energy) and Xue (blood) which flow through distinct meridians (pathways) in the body. When this life force is balanced and circulating properly, the body is healthy. Energy imbalance in the meridians is thought to cause illness or pain. To correct this imbalance, the acupuncturist inserts and stimulates fine needles at acupuncture points.

Acupuncture was developed in China many centuries ago. The Chinese call acupuncture Zhue Jiao, which means "needle heat". The needle regulates an inner force called "Qi", which is responsible for the health of the body. The regulation of Qi using acupuncture can restore physical health, give a release from stress, or improve physical or mental health in other ways. A very healthy person should have Qi energy flowing freely in several distinct pathways, and these pathways are like the roads for maintenance crews. Freely flowing energy distributes everything the cells need, and take away what waste is produced. This produces not only physical, but also mental, health. If Qi is stopped at some point, there will be some symptoms, often a physical illness. The acupuncturist will determine where the needles should be placed in order to return the flow to normal, or as close to normal as is possible. This might happen in one treatment, or a series of treatments. Many

Chinese get acupuncture treatments regularly in order to stay healthy, to keep their Qi flowing at a nearly ideal level. In several places in China, a practitioner of acupuncture gets paid only as long as their clients remain healthy, not when they get sick.

Nearly all acupuncture techniques used needles, though there are varieties that also use electric stimulation, burning, and herbs. The needles used are solid needles, not hollow tube needles like Western doctors use. In America, certified practitioners of acupuncture use pre-sterilized disposable needles. There is usually no medicine on the needles, for the needle itself acts on the Qi energy to make the change in the flow. The practitioner may use a particular angle to insert a needle, or may manipulate the needle a little (such as a small rotation) to get the best results for a particular client.

If you think like the Chinese, you may want to visit your acupuncture clinic regularly to maintain an optimal flow of Qi, and to maintain really good health. A particular health or emotional problem may need only one or two visits, or might require a series of up to eight visits or more, depending on the problem. During a visit, the acupuncturist may insert several needles, and not necessarily at the same points from visit to visit. As the condition improves, a different set of locations might be chosen to affect a change in Qi flow to move even more quickly to good health. Sometimes the needles are inserted just underneath the layer of the skin, while at other times some of the needles may be inserted up to a depth of three inches. Insertion of the needles usually does not hurt at all. Some clients remark on an occasional pinching sensation when a needle is inserted. Once the needle is in place it can easily be forgotten. Sometimes there is a pleasant relaxing or warm sensation around the insertion point, which is an indication that the Qi flow is being redirected in the right manner.

Acupuncture is a very good way to correct a number of illnesses, and one of the best ways to maintain health on a regular basis. This introduction gave a brief overview to encourage you to consider acupuncture as a health option. More and more insurance companies are giving coverage for visits to an acupuncture clinic, and this should be explored.

The Development of Acupuncture

The first known acupuncture text is the Nei Ching Su Wen and there is a great deal of controversy about the exact origins and authorship of this book. The Nei Ching Su Wen is divided into two main sections, the Su Wen, or simple questions and the Ling Shu, or difficult questions. The book is also known by a variety of alternative titles such as the Yellow Emperor's Classic of Internal Medicine, or the Canon of Medicine, but all these titles refer to the same basic text.

Chinese medicine is thousands of years old. The ancient Chinese noticed that certain areas of the skin became more sensitive when a person had a certain health problem. Over time, the Chinese started recording the location of the sensitive areas for a particular symptom or set of symptoms. These areas were associated with the internal organs whose malfunction caused that particular symptom. When outlines of the human body were drawn, these sensitive points were connected in ways to explain the functioning of the human body. The functioning of the body includes the various major organs of the body, and also the entire functional system, including the energy for the organ.

Looking at a text on acupuncture, there will be a number of spots, which relate to the sensitive areas described above. There will also be lines, or "meridians", which connect the various organs and indicate how the energy of the organs flows from one to another. The concept of energy (the "Qi") is fundamental to the application of acupuncture. According to the Chinese, we are given a certain amount of Qi at birth, and this is dissipated by daily living, and restored by ingesting food and air. In the foundation of acupuncture, the imbalance of this energy at various points in the body is the cause of illness. The absence of this energy at some point is death. The Qi circulates through the body in a cycle, moving from meridian to meridian and organ to organ. This energy is constantly moving, dissipating, and being restored.

The use of the needles in acupuncture is to affect the energy level, and so the functioning, of an organ by stimulating or reducing its action. Some organs respond more directly and quickly than others, such as the liver. Acupuncture can be used for pain control, for stress relief, and for a multitude of other physical symptoms and diseases.

China was where the technique of acupuncture and its medical foundations began. Japan also has an extensive history of acupuncture as an accepted and effective treatment for their people. Japanese acupuncture has the same foundations as Chinese acupuncture, but several interesting differences in technique. Acupuncture traveled to Europe in the seventeenth century, being brought back by Jesuit missionaries who had lived in Beijing. Acupuncture did not receive wide acceptance at that point, though there were pockets of practitioners in several places in the West. Acupuncture got significant attention here only when M. Morant from France published many writings on acupuncture in the 1940s. The detail and volume of his writings caught the attention of western physicians, who started considering it for pain control.

The Western doctor observes the facts before him and uses the current physiological theories to explain them. Chinese medicine is based on a much wider world view, which is described in the Nei Ching Su Wen, and these ideas are woven into a complete and intact system based on a philosophy different from that of modern Western medicine. The concepts of Yin and Yang, and the number five, are two of the more important ideas that permeate much of traditional Chinese scientific thought.

Currently, acupuncture is widely accepted by western physicians in several categories, including pain control and stress relief. Indeed, for some operations no anaesthesia is needed at all, just the services of an acupuncturist. This is a distinct advantage, in that the normal operation of the patient's organs is not altered by an artificial anaesthetic. This work in the west has caused new interest and study in the land where acupuncture originated, in China. They have discovered many old, previously unknown texts, and are working on extending the applications. It is an exciting time for the field of acupuncture.

Acupuncture Explained, Eastern and Western

Acupuncture uses the insertion of needles to alleviate certain symptoms in the body. It has gotten wide acceptance among western medicine as treatment for such things as postoperative pain, anesthesia, menstrual cramps, etc. It stimulates a number of points on the body, usually by inserting thin metal needles into points that are carefully selected to address a particular symptom or set of symptoms. When the needles are inserted the patient may feel nothing, may feel more relaxed, or may feel a warm or other pleasant feeling. The reduction of symptoms can occur quite quickly, as in pain release, or over a series of treatments for the symptom.

The Eastern explanation of how acupuncture works comes from China, from a tradition going back more than two thousand years. In this view, the body works best when vital energy circulates around the body exactly as it should. At this time, everything in the body is in balance between two different principles, Yin and Yang. Yin generally is assigned to relaxed, cool, passive objects or feelings. Yang is assigned to active, warm, and assertive objects, organs, and actions. The vital energy flows from one organ system to another to maintain balance between Yin and Yang. When this energy (known as Qi) is blocked or depleted, the body no longer works well and symptoms begin to appear. Qi is assumed to regulate the well-being of the entire person: physical, mental, emotional, and spiritual.

The assumption that Qi regulates all aspects of a person is the reason an acupuncture practitioner easily agrees to treat emotional issues, such as depression and anxiety, with as much enthusiasm as treating physical symptoms. In addition, symptoms that may be a combination of physical, mental, and emotional (such as sleeplessness) fit easily into the acupuncture view of an imbalance of Qi, and are treated accordingly. It also explains why the diagnosis of an acupuncture patient usually includes questions that go well beyond just the physical symptoms of a patient.

Western medicine has been studying the effects of acupuncture with interest for at least the last twenty years. It is clear that there are remarkable successes, and these studies have documented them. However, finding an explanation for the results of a number of these acupuncture studies is a bit more puzzling, if you need an explanation within the western system of medicine. The present view is that the needles affect the behaviour of the nervous system, and stimulation of the system can assist in production of biochemical to produce a particular result. For example, endorphins produced by the body help reduce or eliminate pain, and white blood cells fortify the immune system. However, it is unclear exactly how particular needle stimulation encourages production of particular biochemical. Also, other studies indicate that acupuncture points alter brain chemistry, which affects a number of body functions. This is still a very new and interesting field, and we will continue to see more studies that will help explain the marvellous results of acupuncture technique.

Different Types of Acupuncture Treatment

When you normally think of acupuncture, you think of a person sitting with several needles inserted into their skin, into parts of the body like the ear, the arm, or the wrist. This is a good picture of a patient that is having an acupuncture treatment. These treatments last anywhere from a very short time up to thirty minutes or more, depending on the symptoms that are being treated. These needles are more frequently inserted just far enough into the skin to firmly keep them there, though an acupuncture practitioner may insert different needles somewhat further in depending on the treatment plan. Sometimes the needles are twirled in place; sometimes they are warmed before insertion, or have heat applied to them during insertion. Generally there is no discomfort when a needle is inserted, manipulated, or removed. Occasionally a slight twinge may be felt, but not more than that. Often during treatment a patient may feel more relaxed than when they came in, slightly warmer, or possibly feel a rush of energy during the treatment. Some patients feel no change during the acupuncture treatment, but their symptoms gradually change over a longer period of time, such as several weeks.

Traditional Chinese Medicine is the most common form of acupuncture studied and practiced in the United States. Japanese style acupuncture takes a more subtle route than TCM. Fewer and thinner needles are used with less stimulation. Points in the hand correspond to areas of the body and to certain disharmonies. Points in the ear correspond to areas of the body and to certain disharmonies. This system is commonly used for pain control and drug, alcohol, and nicotine addictions. When a Western Medical Doctor performs Acupuncture; it is defined as Medical Acupuncture. Acupuncture requirements for Western doctors are generally more lenient than for non-Medical Doctor's.

There are variations of acupuncture that do not rely on the use of needles. The ideas behind these are identical with standard acupuncture technique. The knowledge of acupuncture points, the organization of the body, and the importance of proper energy flow for a healthy body are all exactly identical to standard acupuncture therapy. The main difference is that the needle is replaced by a different technique to manipulate the acupuncture point.

In sonopuncture, a device that produces sound waves is applied to the point at which a needle would normally be inserted. In addition to the device that produces the sound waves; other devices that vibrate may also be used, such as tuning forks. There is a good deal of activity in this area, but results using these devices are not as well established as the results with traditional needle based acupuncture.

Another technique that has been in use since the middle of this century is to apply a low voltage electric current to the acupuncture point. Sometimes this is done together with insertion of a needle, sometimes it is done just by touching a small wire to the surface of the skin and connects a very low electric current. The feeling of the current is a very light tingling, and not any very noticeable or painful reaction. This technique using electricity was pursued independently in America and Europe in the 1930s and 1940s, but interest in the technique as a part of western medicine waned after that time.

Another variation of acupuncture that many more people have heard of is the use of acupressure. In this technique no instrument is used, just the technique of pressing a finger on the acupuncture point. This technique can be incorporated into such manipulations as shiatsu massage. This technique is also easy for a layman to do, and many have seen little cards with diagrams of pressure points on the hands and feet. Though these may be useful, the best use is made when the person understands more of the entire system of acupuncture rather than just where the acupuncture points are.

Acupuncture therapy has been extended beyond needles, and interest is continuing in using other instruments. Other techniques include the use of heat (a very traditional choice), friction, magnets, suction, and to the ultra-modern use of laser beams. Acupuncture is a very adaptable therapy, which yields very good results.

Organs in Western and Eastern Medicine

When you visit an acupuncture clinic, you may get treatment and feel much better without ever knowing anything about the philosophy behind acupuncture and that is fine. However, your acupuncture practitioner knows a vast amount of information that is not only interesting, but will help you maintain your health. One area that is particularly interesting is the Eastern medical idea of organs. We all know what organs are, or at least examples of them: heart, liver, lungs, etc. Chinese medicine has a similar concept in several ways, but it looks at them a bit differently. In both views, an organ is a structure that performs certain clearly stated functions. However, in Chinese medicine, each organ also has a particular kind of energy (called Qi) associated with it. This energy flows in certain pathways around the body (called meridians), and so a lot of attention is given to the relation between different organs based on this circulation of Qi. Also, each organ has certain times during the day when it generates a lot of energy, and other times when it is less active. So, an organ is not just a structure, it is a combination structure-energy package that supports and controls the behavior and energy generation of the organs along the energy meridian.

There are twelve organs important to Chinese medicine. The ones that correspond to organs that we are use to include the lung, liver, stomach, heart, and kidney. Western medicine acknowledges the importance of these. Chinese medicine separates out several for individual study: the small and large intestine is two separate organs, and the pericardium (the sac around the heart) is considered a separate organ. Also, the gall bladder and urinary bladder are important in Chinese medicine, less so in western medicine. And finally, there is the "triple warmer" organ, which is a set of three places in the torso that has a particular Qi energy.

The reasons these organs are important to acupuncture is that a healthy body and mind is supported by a normal flow of Qi, and so knowing the locations of the organs and the behavior of the Qi energy is crucial to knowing and re-establishing the normal flow through acupuncture. Centuries of study have associated certain sets of symptoms with dysfunction of a particular organ: for example, dizziness, rib pain, and blurred vision suggest a liver organ malfunction. By listening to physical, mental, and emotional symptoms, and by physical observation of the patient, the acupuncture practitioner can determine the organs that are affected.

An organ may have an excess of Qi energy, or a deficiency. The acupuncture treatment will consist of stimulating the Qi energy flow using needles to rebalance the energy. For example, if an organ has a deficiency, another organ will be designated as a donor organ to supply energy, and so knowing the energy flow between organs is very important. Just like a clogged fuel line, a small change in the delivery system may see a significant improvement in several different places. In this way, a few acupuncture treatments to replenish energy in a particular organ may see improvement in a number of symptoms.

Enjoy your visits to your acupuncture clinic, and the benefits they provide. But remember, there is a world of information that supports these treatments, and knowing more about this is not only interesting, but also helpful in maintaining optimal health.

How Does an Acupuncture Practitioner Diagnose?

Most Americans know that acupuncture has something to do with healing diseases by using needles. These needles are used to redirect and restore optimal circulation of the life force, known as "Qi", within the body. A person with a mental, physical, or emotional problem has the flow of Qi hindered at one or more points, and effective use of needles will change and restore that flow. One of the more surprising things at an acupuncture clinic is the way a problem can be diagnosed. In most cases, the practitioner holds the wrist of the client and takes his pulse. The pulse is observed at several different points on wrist, and the nature of the pulse is evaluated. After that comes a thorough evaluation and a plan of where to place the needles to best address the problem. There are several different qualities the acupuncture practitioner is observing in the pulse.

The patient can have up to 12 different pulse points taken. Three surface pulse points are taken on each of the wrists, and three deep pulse points are also taken on each wrist. Even an untrained person can notice the difference in pulses depending on the location and depth of the pulse point. There are many possible pulse descriptions in acupuncture, but six of the commonly encountered ones are: floating, sunken, slow, rapid, slippery, and choppy. Taking even a few people's pulses, it is easy to see how some could be described as choppy, and others as slippery.

Another very useful technique for diagnosis in acupuncture is by observing the tongue of the client. Western physicians (and mothers!) can often tell someone has a throat problem by looking at the coating on the tongue. But an acupuncture practitioner is looking at a number of aspects of the tongue: the color of the tongue (both top and sides), any cracks that might be in the tongue, swellings, the condition of the dots on the tongue, and the level of moisture. All of these things provide an illuminating picture of the state of someone's health, and indicates what the acupuncture plan should address.

One thing to remember is that, in acupuncture, a particular western medical diagnosis may not be of much help. That is because a particular diagnosis may be caused by one of several different kinds of interruptions in the flow of Qi, and hence is not a major influence in what should be done in the acupuncture clinic. However, the acupuncture practitioner definitely wants to know how you actually feel, for this is very significant. Every symptom should be described, as well as the times they are most noticeable, and any associations that can be thought of. For example, the acupuncture practitioner should be told if pains are milder after a good night's sleep, or if headaches are worse under fluorescent lights, and other such associations.

So expect the diagnosis at an acupuncture clinic to be rather different than a diagnosis at a physician's office. The acupuncture practitioner is not looking just at the particular problem, but how your organs and systems presently interact, one result of which is the current problem. This introduction should make you more comfortable with such a diagnosis, give you more understanding as to why your tongue is being so carefully looked at, and hopefully make you interested enough to find out more about it.

Before you actually receive treatment, the acupuncturist will want to take a history in order to make a clear diagnosis of your condition; this may involve a traditional Chinese history as well as a Western diagnosis depending on the skills and techniques of your acupuncturist. In skilled hands, acupuncture treatment is a relatively painless procedure. You may notice a temporary worsening of your condition, but this usually indicates that an effective response will occur later in the treatment. Treatment usually works in stages, in that the first one or two treatments may produce no effect or perhaps only a transitory effect. A course of six to eight sessions is usually required for effective symptom relief. When such relief has been obtained, it often lasts for three to nine months when one or two further treatments will "top-up" the therapeutic benefit.

When the acupuncture needles are actually inserted, they are usually left in place for between 15 and 30 minutes and often the acupuncturist will try and manipulate the needles so that you will feel a dull bursting or numb sensation around their site of insertion. This sensation is called "de qi" or "obtaining energy" and traditionally it is suggested that "de qi" may be an important part of the treatment process. Sometimes your acupuncturist may use other methods of stimulating the acupuncture point, for instance moxibustion, which is the burning of the herb Artemesia vulgaris just above the surface of the skin or on the end of a needle, or placing a cup over the acupuncture point.

How the Acupuncture Practitioner Uses His Needles

The major focus of an acupuncture treatment is to return the circulation of body energy to its normal levels. To do this, needles are used at points on the body indicated by the set of symptoms for the particular client. These symptoms may be physical, emotional, behavioural, and/or mental. Simply, a needle is inserted at a point in order to either stimulate or dissipate energy. Energy may be dissipated from a point if there is too much activity, which can be indicated by such symptoms as heat or anger. Energy may need to be stimulated by acupuncture if there is seems to be a depletion, as in the case of dizziness or depression.

The points at which needles are to be inserted are determined by an analysis of the client's symptoms, and the organs that are involved in those symptoms. Some change may be affected by simply using pressure on those points (a technique known as acupressure), but far superior results are obtained by being treated by an acupuncture practitioner. There are a number of techniques for using the needles, as well as several different types of needles that can be used. Many modern acupuncture practitioners use small, disposable needles. They can be inserted to different depths, depending on the symptom addressed. It is interesting to compare how the technique to stimulate energy is different than the technique to dissipate energy.

An acupuncture needle used to stimulate energy is sometimes more effective when warmed. The point where the needle is inserted should be massaged before insertion of the needle. Puncture superficially, and then slowly insert the needle to its correct depth slowly, and remove it slowly. The needle should be inserted as the patient exhales, and removed as the patient inhales. The different points should be punctured in the order of energy flow. The needles should remain in place for several minutes, up to ten minutes.

An acupuncture needle used to dissipate energy is rarely warmed, and is inserted and withdrawn rapidly. The needles on average are inserted more deeply than for energy stimulation. The different points should be punctured in the opposite order from the energy flow. The client should inhale as the needle is punctured, and exhale as it is withdrawn. The needle need only remain a few seconds in many cases. Comparing the two techniques, the technique to dissipate energy seems very similar to letting some air out of a balloon or other container: insert quickly and deeply. It is also interesting to note that the patient exhales as the needle is withdrawn, again releasing energy.

The number of needles used varies, but usually 10 to 12 are sufficient. A good acupuncture practitioner never inflicts any pain. At most, there may be a slight feeling of a twinge upon the first insertion, but even that is not to be usual. A needle remaining in the skin is not felt at all as long as it is stationary, and most patients forget about them. There are a number of different kinds of needles, but the only noticeable difference to the client is the difference between a normal needle and a Japanese needle. A Japanese needle is generally thinner and is inside a guide tube, so it will look distinctly different. Needles can come in various widths, with acupuncture needles used for dissipating energy generally thicker than the needles used for energy stimulation.

How Many Acupuncture Treatments Will it Take?

Acupuncture is a well-established and increasingly accepted treatment procedure for pain, for emotional troubles, and for an ever increasing number of physical ailments. More and more traditional physicians are referring patients to acupuncture clinics for a certain set of problems that may be treated more effectively, and without the side effects of medication. Also, individuals may decide to use an acupuncture clinic as the first choice to heal a disease.

The length of a treatment varies widely from person to person, depending on the particular symptoms, the age of the patient, how long the condition has existed, and the environment of the patient. There also seem to be patients that are naturally responsive to acupuncture, when all the other factors are similar. A patient that is responsive to acupuncture may only require one or two visits, as is the case with a number of children. Adult patients that are responsive generally require one to six visits for a particular symptom or set of symptoms. In other cases, up to twenty visits may be required, depending on the severity and length of time the symptoms have persisted. But even some remarkable cases such as recovery from paralysis may come about after a very long series of treatments.

For some conditions, such as for chronic pain, daily treatments are recommended until the pain subsides. The same is true for clients using acupuncture as a means to help stop drug addiction, which require daily treatments in order to keep the cravings at a minimal level. In a few patients, the initial treatment may aggravate the symptoms. A similar possibility is that there is a marked improvement after the first treatment, which may be followed by an aggravation of symptoms at the next few treatments. These should be reported in detail to the acupuncture practitioner, who may revise the locations of needles for the treatment, depending on the particular patient.

It is always a good idea to consider an acupuncture practitioner for whatever health problem you might have. Some problems respond exceptionally well with acupuncture. Acupuncture has a very good success rate for such symptoms as headaches, head congestion, cramps (menstrual, muscular, or intestinal), pain, depression, fatigue, hemorrhoids, and children's nervous disorders. Acupuncture treatments have frequent success in the following areas, though not quite the same success rate as in the areas above. These include diarrhea, painful menstruation, eczema, gastric problems, kidney and gall bladder malfunction, nervous disorders, palpitations, rheumatism, shingles, autonomic nervous problems, especially following surgery.

There are a number of other conditions that acupuncture can be effective for, and for these a practitioner should be consulted, as new results are coming out frequently. Currently, it is thought that acupuncture is more helpful for symptoms rather than curing such diseases as tuberculosis, infantile paralysis, and Parkinson's disease. Acupuncture treatments are sometimes surprisingly effective after traditional medicine has been tried without success. Let's look at two simple cases. In the first, a lady suffered with pain in her ankle for three years, and no standard medical treatment helped. Careful observation of her symptoms by an experienced acupuncture practitioner cured her in three treatments. The second case was of a farmer who had a low grade fever (about 100 degrees) nearly every night for a number of months. Regular physicians could not determine a cause, or a solution. Regular acupuncture treatment was not effective. The acupuncture practitioner then applied the treatments at the optimal time (very early AM, not during the normal clinic hours), and the fever disappeared permanently. I hope this introduction to some uses of acupuncture may help you or someone you know to better health.

After reviewing your medical history, performing an examination, and developing a working diagnosis, your acupuncturist will explain the nature of your condition and his or her recommended treatment plan. The benefits and potential risks of this treatment plan will be explained to you as well as other treatment options as applicable. Depending on the duration, severity and nature of your complaint, the number and frequency of treatments may vary. You may need only one treatment or a series of treatments for more chronic conditions. A typical acupuncture session lasts 30 – 60 minutes. You may be informed that some conditions require coordinated care with other specialists and/or your primary care physician.

A First Visit to an Acupuncture Clinic

You might be thinking about making an appointment at an acupuncture clinic. Many people consider this for various symptoms; some common ones being persistent pain, stress-related symptoms, or other problems such as weight loss. In China, many people use their acupuncture visits as a periodic tune up in order to stay healthy. Chinese acupuncturists sometimes get paid as long as their client is healthy, rather than when their clients have symptoms. So, let us take a tour of a modern American acupuncture clinic to see what it is like.

A typical clinic looks like any professional office, and you will be shown into a room where you are comfortably seated in a chair. The acupuncture practitioner comes in and begins the diagnosis. There are two major parts to the diagnosis, physical observation and a discussion of your symptoms and environment. A basic physical observation will include taking your pulse and observing your tongue. Unlike a traditional doctor's office, your pulse is taken on both wrists, and at several points on each wrist. Your pulse is taken both near the surface of your wrist and also more deeply below the surface. These observations will be written down and used together with the discussion with the practitioner.

You should think about a number of things to discuss at your first acupuncture visit. If you are coming in for a particular symptom or set of symptoms, this should be a major part of the discussion. Think about several different aspects of your symptoms. Let's say that you have persistent pain in your ankle, to use one example. The pain may not be constant during the entire day; it may ebb and wane depending on the hours of the day. The pain may increase or decrease due to certain activities, and you should observe these as much as possible. You might think that walking would certainly increase the pain, but sometimes walking is not as much of a problem as persistent standing, for example, as a cashier in a grocery store. Also, the pain might change depending on the times of the month, and that should also be mentioned to the acupuncture practitioner. Cause and effect, if any, is also important to report. Some things to consider if stress is a component, for possibly the pain started or increased when you got a new supervisor at work. Notice that a diagnosis for an acupuncture visit includes physical, emotional, social, and mental components to the diagnosis. So come to the acupuncture office armed with as much information as you can gather about the reason you are coming.

Once you and the acupuncture practitioner get through the initial diagnosis, sometime is taken to construct a plan of treatments. Depending on the particular symptom that you have, and the other personal information that was taken in the initial diagnosis, your first treatment might be this same day, or you may be asked to return on a different day to start your treatments. The time of day and the particular days for acupuncture treatments are carefully selected in order to achieve the best result possible.

If you do have an initial treatment, it will be painless, and generally takes less than an hour, sometimes much less than that. The acupuncture practitioner will insert very slim needles at specific locations, which will remain for the number of minutes needed for your particular symptoms. When the needles are still you are not even aware of them. Inserting and removing needles is also pain free, rarely there may be a slight twinge, but not more than that. During your treatment you may feel more relaxed a buzz of energy, slightly warmer at the needle insertion points, or exactly the same as when you came in. However, the needles are doing their work to regulate and rebalance the circulation in your body. So enjoy your first visit, and know that each visit brings you closer to your optimal health.

You should be prepared to be comfortable and relaxed for the duration of the treatment. Your acupuncturist may choose various points on your arms, legs, back, or abdomen, so wear loose-fitting clothes, and avoid wearing jewellery, one-piece dresses or tight stockings. Since acupuncture affects your circulation, you will get the most out of a treatment by avoiding heavy meals, alcohol, coffee, or other caffeinated beverages, or participating in rigorous exercise, for about an hour before and after your treatment.

Acupuncture with Herbs

When most people think of acupuncture, they imagine someone sitting in a chair with a number of very thin needles hanging from their ears, or arms, or other parts of their bodies. This is a pretty good picture as far as it goes. The needles are usually not as large as they are imagined to be, and frequently only certain parts of the body have several needles, rather than in a number of different locations.

The purpose of the insertion of the needles is to redirect the flow of energy within the body. Once the flow of energy is restored to its proper channels, the body recovers its proper operation and the systems slowly or quickly disappear. The number of treatments in order for the symptoms to disappear depends both upon the patient and the set of symptoms that are being experienced.

The medical basis for the techniques of acupuncture was developed in China over thousands of years. Part of traditional Chinese medicine also uses a number of herbs, in conjunction with traditional acupuncture technique. In America we are used to taking vitamins and supplements, and we take them as either pills or capsules. Normally we take these supplements as a general nutritional support. The herbs recommended by an acupuncture practitioner are very specific for the symptoms being treated at the clinic. The herbs at the clinic may also be in pills or capsules. They might also be brewed with warm water and taken as a tea. This tea allows the acupuncture practitioner to mix just the right herbs for a particular person, rather than loading them up with several different pills. It is also easier to adjust the proportions in case several different herbs are used. Further, having the herbs taken as a tea makes the action of the herbs very rapid. Your acupuncture practitioner may also offer raw herbs, which have the most potency. They are also the worst tasting choice for someone not used to unusual tastes. However, once raw herbs are tried a few times, most clients prefer the raw herbs.

When your acupuncture practitioner decides on a plan of treatment, you and your practitioner should discuss the various parts of the treatment, including herbs, if any. Remember, not all treatments require herbs, and acupuncture can still be quite effective without them. Make sure that the acupuncture practitioner knows about any vitamin supplements or other nutritional foods presently being used, such as garlic pills or nutritional yeast. Generally nutritional supplements are quite compatible, but it is still important to realize any interactions between regular supplements and the herbs indicated for a particular acupuncture treatment. The same holds true for any prescription medications, even though generally the herbs are not planned to affect a particular organ's mechanism, but rather influence a large part of the body's system as a unit.

Finally, the acupuncture practitioner should be advised of any new symptoms if a new herbal prescription is started. Typically the only symptom might be a slight digestive upset, but if this or any new symptom is noticed, the practitioner should be notified right away. Herbs, though not a necessary part of acupuncture therapy, can be very helpful in promoting more rapid recovery and better health.

Herbal medicine consists mainly of plants, and herbs including roots, barks, flowers, and other natural materials that contain minerals, which help to stimulate the natural healing process of the body. The ingredients are all-natural and contain no synthetic chemicals, hence there are very few side-effect. Each formula (herbal prescription) is tailored to each patient's symptoms. Supplement your diet and balance your nutrition with our natural herbs. Do you know what kind of vitamins and minerals you need? We do and we'll give you all the useful information you can use to get healthy. It's time to think about quality, not the cost.

Acupuncture and Women's Problems

Many of us know about how acupuncture can relieve stress, deaden pain, and be used for other emotional or mental purposes. It is also very useful for a number of problems that women face, from menstrual problems up to the problem of infertility. We will look at a couple of examples to show that acupuncture can be an asset in each case. Of course, you will want to consult your individual acupuncture professional to determine the specific treatment for an individual case.

The first case is a lady with painful and irregular menstrual periods. She gets depressed and irritable, and when she gets angry the pain increases. The first thing to notice about this case is the connection between the cause, menstruation, and the symptoms, which are physical (pain), mental (irritability), and emotional (anger). The acupuncture practitioner is interested in all of these, and symptoms of whatever kind should be reported. Notice also the connection that she sees between increased pain when she is angry, which is also important. A simple analysis of this pinpoints anger and irritability as a log jam of energy in some location in the body. The irregular occasion of the periods suggests the liver. A series of acupuncture visits cleared up the pain and emotional connections to her periods.

A second case is a lady who is going through "the change", and having a hard time with hot flashes and lower back pain. Her acupuncture practitioner talked about the energy around the kidney organ, and that, as we age, there is less kidney energy, and menstruation ceases. The kidney energy has two aspects, Yin and Yang, and hot flashes indicate too much Yang, and the pain in her lower back confirms the Kidney, as that is where it is located. Another common symptom of this, though not in this case, is the symptom of "ringing in the ears". An acupuncture regime for the kidney is prescribed to rebalance the energy and eliminate the symptoms.

The next case is a thirty-six year old woman who cannot conceive. She has already gone through standard western testing, and all hormone levels are acceptable, but nothing has occurred. She normally has somewhat irregular periods, and she is somewhat given to depression. This sounds somewhat similar to the first case because of the irregular periods, and indeed, the liver is included as part of this treatment. Also, from the second case, the kidney energy regulates menstruation, so this organ too is involved in the acupuncture treatment. A second implication of energy problems with the liver is the tendency toward depression.

So, acupuncture has well established treatments for a number of common female problems, and if you suffer from any of these, please asks your acupuncture practitioner. Some of these are treated with more consistent success, for example, the third case illustrated has not yet seen a resolution of her problem. Also notice from the third case, that often western medicine and acupuncture can go hand in hand, as this lady's regular physician had no problem with her seeking a series of acupuncture treatments as a possible solution. One thing that should be emphasized is that the acupuncture treatment is only a manipulation with needles, and involves no medicines whatsoever in these cases. For those of you with menopause or menstruation problems, this has many advantages. Call your acupuncture practitioner.

For most women, breast disease is a very frightening topic, perhaps more so than other life-threatening diseases, such as heart disease. Western medicine has few if any treatments to offer for so-called benign breast diseases. Oriental medicine can diagnose and effectively treat many female breast diseases in their early stages, rather than waiting for Western medical intervention at a later date, which may use radical and invasive procedures. Oriental medicine then can be used as preventive medicine. If a woman has been diagnosed with serious breast disease such as cancer, traditional Chinese medicine in combination with Western medical treatment can be an effective duo to help the individual with emotional issues and easing the harshness of Western treatment.

American society and the media often present menopause, as a disease to be put off as long as possible. From an Oriental medicine perspective, menopause is a naturally occurring transition in women's lives. In many cultures where aging brings power and status, menopausal complaints are almost unheard of. In Western societies where older women are often less valued and respected, around 80 percent of the women have menopausal complaints. Acupuncture is often effective in helping women transition through menopause. From an Oriental medicine perspective, menopausal syndrome often involves the energy of the Liver being stuck and/or a woman's energy (Qi) flowing in the wrong direction. Since a strong point in acupuncture in its ability to regulate energy flow and balancing of the Yin and Yang energies, acupuncture is a well-suited modality for menopausal difficulties. Premenstrual syndrome (PMS) is defined as a collection of differing signs and symptoms, including both mental and physical, which occur only before the menses (after ovulation) and are relieved when menstruation begins. Depending on how premenstrual syndrome is diagnosed, an estimate of women affected with moderate to severe symptoms is about thirty-five percent. PMS has been described as the world's commonest disease.

Acupuncture during pregnancy can be supportive to the woman and fetus in general, but also helpful for some unique and sometimes serious symptoms. With the cessation of the menses, different acupuncture meridians undergo changes which are typical of pregnancy, but do not occur at other times in a woman's life. Commonly acupuncture can often provide relief for morning sickness, edema, anxiety, constipation and other issues for a pregnant woman, as well as support for the woman after delivery. Infertility issues can also be addressed.

Acupuncture and Beauty

Most of us are familiar with the picture of someone getting an acupuncture treatment. We can also list a few things that acupuncture is used for, including reducing anxiety and reducing or eliminating pain. However, few people know that acupuncture is a wonderful thing to add to a beauty routine.

Let us look deeply into the mirror before any makeup is applied. What would we like to get rid of? There are too many fine lines, the dark circles under the eyes are not attractive, and the large pores really should be gone. There is a small hint of a double chin, and the complexion has a few age spots and can't be compared with that of a young woman. Sigh. Well, these things will take a lot of makeup, and maybe more drastic steps, like a little plastic surgery.

Thinking about plastic surgery suddenly makes the thought of a few needles and an acupuncture treatment much easier to tolerate. When an acupuncture practitioner inserts the tiny needles into areas of the face, this stimulates the production of collagen in the general area. The skin will be supported and nourished by the body rather than by some external application. This production of collagen will firm the skin and stretch out any fine lines.

Many women that undergo this procedure have noticed results within one or just a few treatments. Their complexion becomes more even and clear, wrinkles become less noticeable, and there is a general glow to the face. This treatment simply restores the energy of the face to the normal state, and so each woman looks naturally healthier and more beautiful. .Now that our faces our beautiful, we can turn our attention to the rest of our bodies. Most of us have tried, with varying degrees of success, to trim off the extra pounds that we wish were not there. By the time many of us see the wrinkles and dark circles described above visits to the gym no longer produce any truly visible difference.

Successful long term weight loss is incredibly difficult for most of us to achieve. Many people have done all kinds of diets, which just turned into yo-yo dieting. It doesn't seem possible to achieve and keep our weight at a number that is healthy and attractive. This is a second area where acupuncture holds out some promise.

As you would expect, acupuncture weight loss treatment is also done with needles. This time they are not inserted into the face, but instead hair-thin needles are inserted into particular spots on the body that will redirect vital energy to help the body function properly. Sometimes the acupuncture practitioner may also suggest some herbs or an herbal tea. After each acupuncture session is over, most patients feel very good. Western scientists have found that one reason this treatment is successful is the release of endorphins, which is one body chemical that is beneficial in weight loss. The patient continues in a series of treatments, and afterwards maintenance treatments are scheduled periodically. Anyway, healthy people would benefit from a periodic trip to an acupuncture clinic to restore their energy to optimal levels. And these visits will not only keep us healthy, but beautiful as well!

Lucas has been offering this procedure for approximately four and a half years, and last year she began training other acupuncturists in cosmetic acupuncture throughout the United States and Canada. As the procedure gets more publicity, she says, more clients are requesting it, increasing the need for acupuncturists trained in the technique, which requires special acupuncture points and different needling techniques than traditional acupuncture. Cosmetic acupuncture is not for everyone, says Lucas. Though acupuncture has been used to help people with migraines, seizure disorders, or high blood pressure, for example, these people are probably not good candidates for cosmetic acupuncture. For most people, however, Lucas says, acupuncture "lifts" is a great alternative for those who don't want more drastic procedures. Columbia, Md. acupuncturist Della Aubrey-Miller, MAc, LAc, was trained in facial rejuvenation acupuncture, another form of cosmetic acupuncture, which she says is also effective in smoothing out lines, erasing shallow lines, and softening deeper furrows. Still, she says, like surgery, the effectiveness of the treatment depends on what you're starting with. "Working on a 40-year-old face is different from a 60-year-old face," she says. For that reason, both she and Lucas suggest starting the treatments when you're in your 30s, or 40s at the latest.

Acupuncture and Pregnancy

New mothers want the very best for their babies, and this care starts long before the baby is born. Expectant mothers are very careful about nutrition and exercise, and a number of them have started taking regular acupuncture treatments. Treatments are normally scheduled once a month for about forty-five minutes. In the ninth month there is a good deal of preparation for the coming of the baby and preparing the mother for labor, and the treatments are scheduled weekly. The treatments during pregnancy keep the mother in the best health possible, and help quickly disperse any toxins the mother may develop during pregnancy. This keeps the environment in the womb balanced, so that the baby can grow and flourish without complications.

One of the advantages of having acupuncture treatments during pregnancy is the reduction in morning sickness. Studies have shown that women using acupuncture have shorter periods of morning sickness, and they occur less frequently. One of the more common troubles in the second trimester is heartburn, and acupuncture can minimize that symptom also. Even some of the more serious symptoms such as edema and high blood pressure can be treated with acupuncture, but it is important that a physician is also involved in these determinations, as these could be symptoms of major complications. The last trimester has the usual symptoms of backache and joint pain, as the joints loosen in preparation for labor. Acupuncture will address these, and also influence the energy in the mother's body to align the baby properly for delivery.

Acupuncture can also be used in labor, and can also be used to induce labor for women that are overdue. When a mother uses acupuncture to induce labor, frequently there is a distinct feeling of warmth and relaxation. One reason for this is that acupuncture techniques are also able to release stress and anxious feelings, which is a great benefit to the woman facing labor. Compare this feeling to the feeling when a woman is given an injection of oxytocin to start labor. Acupuncture can also be used to increase the energy of the mother during labor.

Once the labor has finished, an acupuncture practitioner's job is not done. Sometimes women bleed after delivery, and insertion of a needle into the proper acupuncture point can stop the blood flow. Several acupuncture treatments over the course of several weeks after delivery can minimize depression, anxiety, and help the body regain its balance more quickly.

More midwives are getting training in acupuncture techniques. Most states have a certification program for acupuncturists, and women considering using acupuncture during their pregnancy should look for this certificate. There is also a certification program nationally for the use of herbs, which is an optional method of treatment in addition to the acupuncture. Many times they go hand in hand, but neither one require the other in order to be effective. Acupuncture is a wonderful tool for the expectant mother, and a well-trained and certified acupuncturist and midwife is a wonderful start for both mother and baby.

Acupuncture as it is practiced today is a safe, comfortable and cost effective treatment for many of the problems that commonly develop in pregnancy. This is especially true since pharmaceuticals are contraindicated in pregnant women in most cases. That being said, it is important to receive acupuncture with a well-trained practitioner because there are some acupuncture points that are traditionally forbidden to do during the nine months of gestation. These points are the ones that are known to strongly move Qi (energy) and blood through the pelvis, including obvious points like those on the lower abdomen, and also the famous points we use to treat gynaecological disorders: LI4 and SP6. In fact these two points when strongly stimulated have been used to induce abortion. Acupuncture, of course, when properly applied can help to prevent, not cause miscarriages.

Acupuncture and Electricity

Acupuncture has been shown to have great success in treating pain, stress, and a number of diseases. Acupuncture has a number of different techniques, and one of them is to apply a very low-level electric charge to the needle. This particular technique is creating interest in a field that was started in America in the 1930s and 1940s, but lost support soon afterward. This field is how to use low levels of electricity as a tool for medical therapy.

The initial discovery of acupuncture points on the body was by centuries of observation of the tender spots on the skin when a patient had certain symptoms. These acupuncture points can now be discovered and duplicated by scientists. They can find these same acupuncture points (given in any standard diagram) by using electrical apparatus. Scientists can also use infrared photography to find the temperature differences between these acupuncture points and the surrounding skin. So the acupuncture points have a different electrical behavior than the surrounding cells when the patient suffers from the associated symptom.

Several claims for acupuncture seem to get some support from other research using electricity. One scientist, Becker, has had tissue regrown by animals when he applied a low-level electric current to the site of the tissue. Even heart tissue has been restored without any scarring. Low level electric pulses have also been used to make bone fractures heal significantly faster than fractures left to heal on their own.

How do these two previous experiences relate to the fundamentals of acupuncture? The basis of acupuncture is the correct distribution and flow of energy throughout the body. When energy is depleted, regrowth and stimulation and vitality do not occur. An acupuncture treatment restores the energy needed to a specific area. This research (especially the bone research) supports the claim that acupuncture sessions are of significant benefit for those with broken arms or other broken bones in the feet, ankles, and wrists, or other locations. Acupuncture has been known as an effective treatment for patients with heart palpitations, and the EKG results scientifically support that claim.

When an acupuncture needle is inserted into the skin, there is an electrical activity at that point, since the cells at that point are disturbed, and cells by their structure have various electrical charges within them. This is also shown by such techniques as Kirlian photography, where the photograph after a needle is inserted has a very different energy shape than before the needle insertion.

This exploration of the interaction between electricity and acupuncture has come back to expand the techniques used in acupuncture. The most basic technique for an acupuncture treatment is to use needles inserted into the skin of the patient. The location of the insertion, its depth and technique, bring about the results from the treatment. An additional technique is the application of heat, or moxa, which we will not go into. A third addition may be the use of herbs, either at the point of insertion, or given to the patient separately. A technique directly related to the above research, and also harkening back to the experiments of the 1930s and 1940s, is to affect the acupuncture points by a low voltage electric current. This is used in place of the needle. All these results and new ideas make research in acupuncture an exciting field to be working in and reading about.

The electro-acupuncture device is not intended to provide a significant current between the acupuncture needles. Rather, it delivers about 10-80 milliamps depending upon the selected setting. But, it will provide a significant voltage: 40-80 volts, which is the basis for the patient response. In the commonly-used portable battery devices, this is accomplished by boosting the voltage output of the battery, such as raising the voltage from 9 volts to 45 volts. Many of the devices have an AC adapter to avoid frequent replacement of batteries, and this involves a substantial step-down of both voltage and amperage. There is virtually no current transmitted through the body, but there is enough voltage stimuli for the patient to feel it; often this will be a pulsating sensation because of the intention of using a waveform that is perceptible. Duration of standard treatment with electro-acupuncture is usually 10-20 minutes and rarely exceeds 30 minutes.

The electrical pulsing stimulus is used in a few cases for an hour or more, especially for difficult to treat neurological disorders. During the stimulation period, the patient may become adapted to the stimulus (this will typically happen after the first minute or two), with a gradual decline in response. The electrical output should then be adjusted in frequency and/or intensity to resume the sensation. Variable frequency output of the electro-acupuncture device is sometimes utilized in an attempt to circumvent this adaptation. Electro-acupuncture is normally administered with alternating current. Therefore, the two electrodes in any pair are equivalent, even if they are color coded to distinguish them. Some devices allow a direct current (non-alternating) setting, but the use of this has been discouraged, as mild adverse effects might occur if the pulsing of the current ceases for any reason (i.e., device defect). Further, it has been suggested, though it remains to be proven, that the adaptation to the direct current may be more rapid than to the alternating current.

A device commonly used in China is the G6805 or G6805-2 electric stimulator. The device should not be turned on until after the acupuncture needles are in place and the electrodes connected. All changes in the electrical stimulus should be carried out gradually. It is normal for the patient to experience responses such as rhythmic spasm or weak twitching of the muscle (frequently visible to the practitioner), as well as the usual "deqi" reactions of acupuncture therapy: sensation of numbness, distension, and/or heaviness. The stimulus intensity, set by a voltage-adjusting knob on the device, should be in the range between the minimum amount needed for the patient to sense its effect and the minimum amount that produces an uncomfortable reaction; care should be taken to limit the muscle twitching to a mild response. Areas that are particularly sensitive to electrical stimulation are the face and regions below the elbow and knee. These areas should be treated initially with a very low intensity voltage. Patients who have not had acupuncture previously should receive standard acupuncture first to assure that they tolerate the treatment well, before moving on to electro-acupuncture, which may yield a stronger sensation.

Although some theories have been developed regarding the mechanism of action of electro-acupuncture, there are no conclusive tests. The main function of electro-acupuncture, as evidenced by the discussions in several clinical reports in the Chinese medical literature, appears to be no more than pulsation by voltage spikes serving as stimulus replacing a rhythmic physical movement as stimulus at the site.

Acupuncture and Drug Abuse

Acupuncture is a bright light on the road to recovery for many drug addicts and alcoholics. As an addict is recovering, the physical and psychological urge to get another fix or get another drink can be overwhelming. If the addict can get past that feeling, there is more hope for another successful day on the road to recovery. Currently there are a number of chemicals to help reduce that feeling, such as the nicotine patches to help people stop smoking. However, a major advantage of using acupuncture is that it uses no chemicals in the treatment, can be used for a number of different addictions, and is quite inexpensive compared to a number of other treatments.

Let's take a look into a clinic that uses acupuncture to treat recovering addicts. Before the clinic used acupuncture, it was somewhat loud and not a pleasant place to be. The treatment room holds dozens of clients at the same time, each sitting in a chair. Each person sits with five long needles dangling from each ear. Depending on the person, a few also have some acupuncture needles in their hands, arms, or feet. When the time comes to remove the needles, some are removed by one of the acupuncture practitioners, or an assistant, or some clients remove their own needles at the appropriate time. Needles are left in the patient for an average of about forty-five minutes. The chairs are arranged so that the clients can see and talk to each other if they wish. This helps when they share experiences, and helps if some of the new clients are nervous about the use of acupuncture. The room, though it holds a number of often troubled patients, is generally quite calm and peaceful.

What advantage is there in using acupuncture for a recovering addict? Most of the addicts describe a release of that feeling that insists they must find a fix or must find a drink. The patient describes it as the feeling when you get home after a long day and take off your shoes. The effect of the treatment lasts for about a day, and so newly recovering addicts are scheduled for daily treatments. People such as dry alcoholics can come by on a periodic basis, or when they feel they need another acupuncture treatment. Many dry alcoholics are fine as long as their daily life is not stressful, but if a family problem arises at home or at work, the familiar feeling becomes strong once again. At those times an acupuncture clinic is a great help, for it affects an actual physical change in the person.

Many detox clinics that use acupuncture in its regimen incorporate it into an overall program, where the acupuncture treatments are the first steps that a patient takes. A typical clinic will schedule a new patient for daily acupuncture sessions, and at each session take a sample to ensure the patient has not used drugs during the past day. After 10 "clean" days, the patient is considered in sufficient shape to start additional therapy, such as a twelve step program. Acupuncture treatments continue during this time. If a patient has a relapse, the patient just starts all over again with the ten day acupuncture treatment.

Using acupuncture in recovery programs has definite advantages, both economically and in support of physical and mental health for the recovering addicts. It is just another example where the use of acupuncture incorporates healing in all areas: physical, mental, and emotional.

What advantage is there in using acupuncture for a recovering addict? Most of the addicts describe a release of that feeling that insists they must find a fix or must find a drink. The patient describes it as the feeling when you get home after a long day and take off your shoes. The effect of the treatment lasts for about a day, and so newly recovering addicts are scheduled for daily treatments. People such as dry alcoholics can come by on a periodic basis, or when they feel they need another acupuncture treatment. Many dry alcoholics are fine as long as their daily life is not stressful, but if a family problem arises at home or at work, the familiar feeling becomes strong once again. At those times an acupuncture clinic is a great help, for it affects an actual physical change in the person. Many detox clinics that use acupuncture in its regimen incorporate it into an overall program, where the acupuncture treatments are the first steps that a patient takes. A typical clinic will schedule a new patient for daily acupuncture sessions, and at each session take a sample to ensure the patient has not used drugs during the past day. After 10 "clean" days, the patient is considered in sufficient shape to start additional therapy, such as a twelve step program. Acupuncture treatments continue during this time. If a patient has a relapse, the patient just starts all over again with the ten day acupuncture treatment. Acupuncture is widely accepted by medical professionals in the United States as a safe treatment for chronic pain. Other applications for acupuncture, such as relief of asthma, arthritis, nausea, and morning sickness are being explored by the scientific community.

In the case of drug addiction, conclusive scientific evidence of acupuncture's efficacy is scarce. A 1989 study published in the British journal The Lancet by Milton L. Bullock concluded that acupuncture was highly effective in treating alcoholism. Eighty severe recidivist alcoholics were treated, receiving either correct-point acupuncture or acupuncture at non-specific points on the ear. 21 of the 40 treatment group patients completed the two-month program, while only one of 40 in the control group did. The control group patients experienced twice as many relapses in the six months following the experiment and the number of control group patients admitted to detoxification centers was well over twice that of treatment group patients.

Acupuncture and Children

As parents, we all want our children to be happy and healthy. Consider the idea that acupuncture might be a wonderful way to treat your child's health. Acupuncture can be good preventative treatment, as well as a technique to cure various symptoms. In China, some acupuncture professionals in China are paid only as long as their clients remain healthy!

Your first question might be if any children are actually acupuncture clients? Sure! Nearly all children find acupuncture treatments very easy, even enjoyable. Especially the younger ones, for acupuncture needles are not painful, and younger children don't have our "a needle is painful" association that adults do. Children also seem to be more aware of their bodies than adults, and can feel themselves feeling better quite quickly. Also, the improvement in energy and vitality is often so clear with children.

Are there differences for acupuncture treatment with children? The general treatment is similar, determining the locations and times to insert needles in order to effect the treatment. (Needles are inserted to different depths depending on the treatment, anything from just under the skin up to a maximum of a few inches. Even so, the needle insertion does not hurt. Sometimes an insertion can be described as a "slight pinch", but once the needle is in, it isn't felt at all unless it is moved.) The number of needles and the number of treatments for children is generally less, for their very active bodies respond quickly to less stimulation. Because of this, acupuncture treatments for children often bring noticeable results very quickly.

Another good reason to visit an acupuncture clinic with your child is that the diagnosis uses a number of different aspects: physical symptoms, observed physical signs such as the pulse and condition of the tongue, behavioral symptoms such as anger, aggression, depression, an even external physical conditions and the time of year. A goal of acupuncture is to bring the whole person into harmony: physically, emotionally, mentally, and socially. This attention to the child as a whole is of great benefit, both to the child and to your whole family.

You can bring your child in for an acupuncture visit to maintain their health, for a physical symptom, or for a behavioral problem. One common problem that frequently responds quite well to several acupuncture visits is the problem of bed-wetting. Some children have the problem disappear after one acupuncture visit; others may require a few more visits. Interestingly, most parents are aware that the child has negative emotions, and assume that of course it stems from having wet the bed. However, a number of parents report that, after thinking on it, that actually sadness or other emotion preceded the bedwetting by several weeks. This is not always true, but there is often a connection other than the assumed "wet the bed then feel bad" connection.

Something that you may want to discuss with your acupuncture practitioner is child vaccinations. As time goes on, more vaccines seem to become available for a wider range of diseases, as the recent popularity of the chicken pox vaccine. Most acupuncture practitioners have a list of vaccines they still strongly recommend, such as the vaccine against polio. It is worthwhile to discuss the various vaccines with your acupuncture practitioner.So, please consider an acupuncture practitioner as a wonderful health specialist for your child. Children's bio-energetic systems are not fully formed and, being at the most "yang" phase of their existence, their energy (Qi) moves extremely rapidly. Consequently, children's systems can be easily over stimulated, and health problems can progress rapidly. Shonishin focuses on gentle, specialized, mostly non-inserted treatment techniques that children find comfortable and even pleasurable. Dramatic results can be obtained even with very light treatment.

The ancient classics of China, such as the Ling Shu, describe nine types of needles, several of which were clearly never intended to pierce the skin. Three of these non-inserted needles — the enshin, the teishin, and the zanshin — are considered basic to the practice of shonishin pediatric acupuncture. Over the years, many additional tools and supplementary techniques have been designed specifically for pediatric therapy. Shonishin techniques involve rhythmic stroking, rubbing, tapping, and pressing the skin to give different kinds of gentle stimulation. These techniques harmonize and fortify the child's vital energy, and strengthen the child's constitution.

Acupuncture and Biorhythm

We all know something about biorhythms. Basically, a biorhythm is an internal clock that regulates our bodies in relation to the daily positions of the sun, and the monthly positions of the moon. This can be seen in the time it takes our bodies to adjust to small changes, such as the changes of daylight savings time, or in large changes, such as jet lag. Our understanding of and interest in biorhythms has been recent, within the last thirty or forty years.

The ancient Chinese observed this connection between our bodies and the planets many centuries ago, and use it in their practice of acupuncture. They list a number of different biorhythms, from the normal twenty four hour cycle up through longer several day periods. All of these are used to follow and influence fluctuations in body energy.In acupuncture, this energy circulates through each part of the body throughout the day, each organ having a two hour time for maximum energy and a time for minimum energy. For example, the major organs have their maximum energy in the following order: first the liver, then the lungs, large intestine, stomach, spleen, heart, etc., in sequence, for all of the twelve major organs. This order was discovered by years of observing the times of day that the disorders of the various organs displayed their worst symptoms. The acupuncture practitioner can use the times of a patient's symptoms to help determine which organs and energy channels are affected, and also help select the favorable times to treat the patient. For example, many of the worst asthma attacks take place during the wee hours, which is the maximum energy period of the lungs. The best time to treat these cases is at a time or as close to the time as possible.

In the science behind acupuncture, a symptom may be caused by too much energy at an organ, and other symptoms by an insufficient amount of energy. (The determination of which symptoms fall into which category has been catalogued over many centuries, and there are many books on acupuncture detailing these for each of the major organs.) The best time to treat a symptom associated with too much energy is during its maximum energy output, and a symptom with a deficiency in energy is just after the maximum output is over. Of course, it may not be possible to get to your practitioner at those particular times, and there are also other good choices at other times of the day.

In addition to the daily biorhythm, there are also ten day intervals associated with the moon, and so the acupuncture practitioner might strongly suggest that a particular day would be better for treatment than another, based on the particular symptoms reported. Each day of the ten days is associated with one of two aspects of the Qi energy, and also associated with one of five elements. Particular organs are associated with particular elements, and so stimulation of these organs will be more successful on those days associated with the correct element.

It is important for us to take note of the times our symptoms occur as well as what our symptoms are, for that is important information in our acupuncture treatment plan. And know that the time and dates for our treatments are an important part of how well the treatment works.

Stress, High Blood Pressure, and Acupuncture

When a person is under stress, their body starts what is known as a stress response. A number of chemicals are released into the bloodstream, the heart beats faster, breathing becomes more rapid, and muscles tense up. If the person is planning on running away from a large animal, these are all very good responses. For the businessman at his desk taking a phone call, these are not good reactions. The body easily takes care of an occasional response like this, the chemicals are cleaned out, and the body becomes relaxed once again. However, when this reaction occurs a number of times a week, the stress starts to affect the resting state of the body. Muscles no longer entirely relax, and the frequent release of these chemicals creates other problems. Chronic stress can cause such problems as sleeplessness, stomach and digestion problems, panic attacks, and pain of some sort (such as frequent headaches). Long term problems related to stress include strokes, high blood pressure, and colitis or other bowel problems.

A person may try to handle stress on his or her own, by finding something to mask it. Alcohol, caffeine, cigarettes, and even lots of sugar can make the person feel better. Onc of the most common "pills" after a stressful moment is a cup of coffee and a doughnut, or possibly a cigarette. Physicians can also prescribe medications to combat some of these symptoms, both psychological and physical. Antidepressants, one of the more common medications for this, only offer short-term relief at best.

The obvious answer is to remove the source of stress. However, many times that simply is not possible. Is there another solution? One of the most successful results from acupuncture is the relaxation of the patient, followed by the removal of tension from the body. This relaxation response produces a decreased heart rate, lowered blood pressure, and increased energy and possible tissue regeneration. There is frequently a feeling of well-being and self-confidence. As the acupuncture treatment stimulates and redirects the vital energy of the body, each muscle and organ system begins to function the way that it should. Acupuncture is not only used to relieve the stress response of a patient, but also in a number of cases it has made the doctor prescribed antidepressant unnecessary. With wider use of acupuncture, there could be a substantial reduction in the consumption of drugs such as Prozac.

Standard acupuncture techniques using needles are very effective to combat chronic stress. If this were more widely accepted by Americans under routine stress, we would have a much healthier population. In addition, acupuncture treatments that use low levels of electricity have been found to be even more successful in lowering blood pressure. Several researchers that use electric stimulation have been able to regrow tissue in animals without any scars. The combination of using acupuncture therapy for blood pressure management and possible healthy tissue regrowth is a very exciting topic for people with heart and circulatory problems

Acupuncture is one of the most successful treatments for this American problem. Not only do the symptoms decrease, but the acupuncture treatment results in a healthier body as well.

Acupuncture and Extreme Cases

What are some extreme cases where acupuncture is useful? Let us talk about a few particularly interesting ones. The first is using acupuncture on a person in a coma. Many times people in comas only receive minimal care. When my father was in a long term care hospital, I often walked by two rooms where the occupants were in comas, one I knew had been that way for at least several months. After treating any conditions that the doctors were aware of, there was little else to do for these patients. The one that was there for months never had any visitors as far as I could see, and the hospital was maintaining him until at some time he might come out of his coma. The practice of acupuncture can help a person in a coma in the following ways: clear the physical senses, calm the spirit, clear the brain, strengthen the heart, and eliminate phlegm. Without getting too specific, these areas are regulated by different organs of the body and the energy from those organs, and insertion of needles at correct points will redirect that energy.

Depending on the patient, sometimes the needles might be twirled gently. Western medicine distinguishes comatose patients based on their originating symptom (brain tumor, car accident, etc), but the practice of acupuncture groups the patients by their set of common symptoms. The use of acupuncture for these patients will improve their overall well-being, and in some cases the patients revive after a time, though it is not possible medically to determine why they revive.

A second use of acupuncture is for someone that is prone to simple fainting. As a caution, a physician should determine if the cause is serious heart trouble. If not, there are standard acupuncture regimes which will regulate energy to allow the blood to freely recirculate through the entire body, including the head. It is also interesting to note that a number of times this physical symptom can be accompanied by a social problem such as overwork, or an emotional problem such as internally rebelling from a situation that the patient wanted to be released from. Acupuncture can restore harmony to both the physical and emotional components of the patient.

Another application of acupuncture is for patients in emergency situations. It would be best to have an actual acupuncture practitioner at the scene, but anyone can use these simple techniques. If someone has lost consciousness, apply a strong pressure with your fingernail in the groove between the nose and mouth, about one third of the way down from the nose. This is a simple acupuncture point that may well awaken the patient. Chest-related emergencies can be helped with the acupuncture point on the underside of the forearm, between the two tendons, and about two thumb widths back from the last wrist crease. This may help for people experiencing palpitations, hiccups, stomach pain, and lung problems. Press firmly.

These just list a few unusual applications where acupuncture would be useful. There are also acupuncture regimens for people that have gone into shock, a drowning victim that is now breathing but still unconscious, acupuncture support for patients with broken limbs, etc. I hope this has expanded your view on many additional uses for acupuncture.

A Personal Experience with Acupuncture

Let's follow Susan as she goes to her first acupuncture treatment. Susan is a little hesitant, thinking of many needles sticking out of her in funny places so that she can't find a place to sit easily. Her friend Marie had recommended this acupuncture clinic as a possible help for Susan's recent problems of sleeplessness and depression. Susan was very surprised that Marie had ever visited an acupuncture clinic, as Marie didn't seem to be someone that would visit something this unusual. And anyway, Marie always seems so remarkably healthy, attending the gym on a regular basis and still having lots of energy to spare. Susan was surprised to find out that Marie had been going to this acupuncture clinic for more than three years. She was even more surprised to find out that the first visit was suggested by Marie's doctor - her family physician. Susan had no idea that a regular doctor would recommend a visit to an acupuncture clinic.

It turns out that a few years ago Marie had very intense cramps, and after a discussion with her doctor, they decided acupuncture might help to reduce or eliminate these. After having that treatment, Marie had discovered that some people visit the acupuncture clinic periodically just to keep in good health. Marie really enjoyed the way she felt, and so continued with the periodic visits as a kind of "tune up," as she called them.

Though this is Susan's first treatment at the acupuncture clinic, it is her second visit. Her first visit was to sit with the acupuncture practitioner to take several vital signs and to have a long discussion about her symptoms. Susan explained that she was hoping to get relief from the sleeplessness and depression through the treatments at the acupuncture clinic. She was surprised at the number of questions that she hadn't thought about. She hadn't noticed if the sleeplessness was the same on every night, or if she got to sleep more easily on some nights. She hadn't noticed if she easily returned to sleep if she was awakened once she was asleep. She hadn't thought about whether the sleeplessness started after they turned off the central heat in the house, now that spring had come. There were so many questions about that. There were questions she had expected, like that her depression could be related to the fact that her best friend at work had left for a new job. There were also surprising questions about patterns that she noticed about any previous depressions that she might have had. Once all the questions had been answered, Susan was asked to return another day for her first treatment in order to obtain the most beneficial results.

Susan pulled into the parking lot, still a little nervous. The acupuncture practitioner was a very nice and calm woman, but still... Twenty minutes later, Susan was sitting in a comfortable chair with about 18 needles at various points on her arms and ears. She was very comfortable, and inserting the needles did not hurt at all. After sitting there for 15 minutes, the acupuncture practitioner came in, removed the needles and that was it. Susan was amazed! A sequence of 6 treatments had been prescribed initially, and they agreed to revisit Susan's symptoms when these were done. She was so happy it was so easy!

Another story is of a person named David. I have been suffering from haemorrhoid, hemafecia, and prolapse of anus for a long time. Upon the suggestion of a western physician, I had a surgery to end these diseases. The surgery did a wonderful job in getting rid of my above health problems. Nevertheless, I cannot forget two episodes caused by the side effects of my surgery. Due to my age and the strong effect of anaesthesia, I had retention of urine after the surgery. From the early morning when I had the surgery till the midnight, not a single drop of my urine could come out. Fortunately, I was hospitalizing for observation by then. After contacting the doctor, the nurse used intubation for catheterization and I left the hospital the next day.

In the third day, I went to the hospital for return visit, the doctor removed the tube and told me that everything was fine and I could take some antiphlogistics. After another day, however, I could not urinate again. I felt so bad that I had to contact the doctor. He had no other solutions except suggesting me to have fomentation. I followed his instruction but it did not work. One of my friends suggested me to visit Dr. Kexin Bao. I did. Dr. Bao thought it was caused by a problem in the nerve and acupuncture did extremely well in dealing with problems of this kind. He selected several points in my lower abdomen and put the needles at these places. Over half an hour, he removed the needles. Just after the treatment, I could urinate. It was really magical!

The second problem I had after the surgery was constipation. Following the doctor's suggestion, I took medicine on time each day, took a shower at a sitting position, had cellulose food and drank some special made fruit juice, but none of them made effect. I had consulted the doctor; the medicine he prescribed was the same as before. Had I taken his prescription again constipation would have persisted and I could not bear it any more. What could I do?

Then I remembered the experience I had last time (my inability to urinate). So I visited Dr. Bao. He gave me acupuncture again. As before, he cured my disease. When I returned home the same afternoon, I had no problem in defecation. To be honest, I knew little about medicine. But through my above personal experience, I realize profoundly the importance of urination and defecation is to our health. I also profoundly realize that Chinese acupuncture has its unique curing effect which is lack in western medicine, especially on its excellent effect. It can cure these diseases almost with the point of the needle. Of course, most importantly, no matter how well the medical skills can be, only when they are used by good doctors with medical ethics, can they have been achieved their functions. Any bogus art of healing will not help curing any disease. Here I would like to end my article by saying from the bottom of my heart: "Thank you, Dr. Bao!"

Yin and Yang and Acupuncture

The ancient Chinese considered harmony to be the goal of our lives as individuals, and also as a society. When harmony is disturbed in our physical or emotional lives, it is restored by the use of acupuncture. Harmony is a continual balancing act between opposites: opposites in color, in energy, in actions, etc. This idea of opposites is seen even in the west with such ideas as positive and negative ions in chemistry and physics. The Chinese denote the opposite ends of each idea as "yin" and "yang". They are not opposed to each other, but are the ultimate in each direction. For example, rest is Yin and exercise is Yang, or Yin is cold winter and Yang is hot summer. Life would not be in balance if it were entirely exercise or entirely rest, and so balance of Yin and Yang produces harmony. Notice that Yang is the active, warm, excitable, aggressive side, whereas the corresponding opposite Yin is restful, cool, calming, and passive.

Acupuncture is concerned with the optimal flow of the energy Qi. Harmony is disturbed by a lack of balance, and a lack of balance will constrict or overemphasize the flow of Qi at various points in the body. The acupuncture practitioner has four sets of diagnostic features, each of which have a yin end and a yang end. Three of these are specific: hot and cold, interior and exterior, and excess and deficiency. So, for example, someone who spends all of their time inside eating sweets has at least two imbalances that can be noted by the acupuncture practitioner. There is also a fourth, general set, for any other features that should be noted in the acupuncture diagnosis that are not covered by the first three: for example, an unusually passive person. A harmonious personality should have a balance between aggressiveness and passivity, each at the appropriate times.

It may be surprising that the treatment of acupuncture takes mental and emotional states into account, but the goal of acupuncture is to restore harmony to the whole person. A number of imbalances may not have caused a physical health problem, but rather such symptoms as strife within the family, a tendency to cry easily, or other social or emotional symptom. These are strong indicators and also need to be addressed.

The goal of is to restore harmony and redirect Qi energy to its normal flow. This energy is active and always moving, and hence has Yang qualities. So, if you were an acupuncture practitioner and had a client who noticed they were being unusually aggressive and angry lately, you would suspect a buildup in energy at some organ in the body. Whereas, if someone were depressed and listless, that would be an indication of a deficiency of energy at some organ or organs in the body. This, along with a diagnosis of physical symptoms, would give the best acupuncture treatment to address this.

So, by organizing objects, actions, conditions, and other attributes of life into "Yin" and "Yang", the acupuncture practitioner can more easily fit mental, social, and emotional issues into the overall treatment plan for each of the clients. The method of acupuncture is to restore the normal flow of Qi, which in turn will restore harmony and balance into the patient's life.

Acupuncture's Acceptance in America

Acupuncture has been used in China and Japan for centuries, and was introduced into Europe in the 1700s by Jesuit missionaries. However, it has been popular in the United States for only the past twenty or thirty years. Initially, its most dramatic and effective results here in America were to reduce or eliminate pain, where some patients undergoing surgery had no anesthesia whatsoever. Their pain was eliminated during the surgery by use of acupuncture needles.

The National Institute of Health has been interested in both the use and the growing interest in acupuncture, and has had a number of conferences whose main subject is the use of acupuncture. Interestingly, thousands of traditional physicians, dentists, and other health practitioners now use acupuncture for pain relief and other symptoms. Also, currently more than 10 million adults in the U.S. have used acupuncture at some time in the past, or are using it currently. (Though acupuncture is also perfectly safe for children, and frequently children respond more quickly to the treatments than adults.)

The National Institute of Health has looked at many studies on the effectiveness of acupuncture to relieve a specific set of symptoms. There are some outstanding successes, but making any sweeping statement is difficult because many of the studies are not easy to design. Or, more properly, there is some heated discussion on what studies have been so carefully designed that the results are beyond question. But there is general agreement that acupuncture is highly effective for a wide range of symptoms, including pain and nausea after operations, headaches, menstrual cramps, asthma, osteoarthritis, etc. Research is continuing and new results are coming out quite often. One of the best ways to keep up is to search the Internet for your symptom of interest together with the key word "acupuncture". Also look for websites sponsored by NCCAM, a branch of the National Institute of Health that investigates alternative medicines.

Since the main equipment of an acupuncture practitioner is needles, the needles in an acupuncture office are regulated by the government to ensure safety of the needles. The FDA approves their use by licensed practitioners in acupuncture clinics. The requirements are that the needles are sterile needles and one time use only, so no one need be concerned about the problem with needle contamination. The acupuncture needles are regulated by the same rules as those in your doctor's office. To avoid any concern, watch carefully that the acupuncture practitioner opens a new, sealed package for each patient and swabs the insertion sites with some kind of disinfectant before inserting the needle (such as alcohol, traditionally used by nurses).

Acupuncture has evolved from an interesting import from China to an established technique that many doctors recommend, or has even become trained in the technique themselves. Acupuncture clinics and practitioners now have standards set up and regulated by the government in order to ensure the safety of the clients. It has become an accepted part of the mainstream American health system. The National Institute of Health has been interested in both the use and the growing interest in acupuncture, and has had a number of conferences whose main subject is the use of acupuncture. Interestingly, thousands of traditional physicians, dentists, and other health practitioners now use acupuncture for pain relief and other symptoms. Also, currently more than 10 million adults in the U.S. have used acupuncture at some time in the past, or are using it currently.

The National Institute of Health has looked at many studies on the effectiveness of acupuncture to relieve a specific set of symptoms. There are some outstanding successes, but making any sweeping statement is difficult because many of the studies are not easy to design. Or, more properly, there is some heated discussion on what studies have been so carefully designed that the results are beyond question. But there is general agreement that acupuncture is highly effective for a wide range of symptoms, including pain and nausea after operations, headaches, menstrual cramps, asthma, osteoarthritis, etc.

Research is continuing and new results are coming out quite often. One of the best ways to keep up is to search the Internet for your symptom of interest together with the key word "acupuncture". Also look for websites sponsored by NCCAM, a branch of the National Institute of Health that investigates alternative medicines. Since the main equipment of an acupuncture practitioner is needles, the needles in an acupuncture office are regulated by the government to ensure safety of the needles. The FDA approves their use by licensed practitioners in acupuncture clinics. The requirements are that the needles are sterile needles and one time use only, so no one need be concerned about the problem with needle contamination. The acupuncture needles are regulated by the same rules as those in your doctor's office. To avoid any concern, watch carefully that the acupuncture practitioner opens a new, sealed package for each patient and swabs the insertion sites with some kind of disinfectant before inserting the needle (such as alcohol, traditionally used by nurses).

This survey is intended to give an overview of how the traditional medical community and also the institutes of the government have given credibility to the use of acupuncture. Acupuncture has evolved from an interesting import from China to an established technique that many doctors recommend, or have even become trained in the technique themselves. Acupuncture clinics and practitioners now have standards set up and regulated by the government in order to ensure the safety of the clients. It has become an accepted part of the mainstream American health system.

The American Academy of Medical Acupuncture

It is surprising to many people that a large and growing number of traditional physicians support the use of and practice of acupuncture techniques. The American Academy of Medical Acupuncture was organized by physicians who want to further the use of acupuncture in regular medical treatment. The Academy was founded nearly twenty years ago by a group of physicians trained in acupuncture, which graduated from courses sponsored by the UCLA School of Medicine. It used to be that acupuncture practitioners had vast knowledge of the traditional acupuncture techniques and philosophy, but little or no training in traditional western medicine. At the other end of the medical spectrum were physicians, who knew nothing about traditional Chinese medicine, and looked with some doubt on the claims of acupuncture treatment. However, a number of studies and experiments showed that acupuncture gave consistently good results in a number of areas, and so physicians started referring their patients for particular problems, such as persistent pain. After some time, traditional physicians starting learning and using acupuncture techniques as part of their own methods of treatment. In addition to the techniques, they learned the long history behind the current acupuncture techniques.

The Academy (known as AAMA) is important to both physicians and patients, for members of the AAMA meet the highest standards for both traditional medicine and certified acupuncture practitioners. Most patients implicitly trust physicians, both for their extensive training and for their high standards of practice. They extend both of these to the practice of acupuncture within their offices.

One of the goals of the AAMA is to spread knowledge and appreciation of acupuncture to other physicians and health professionals that presently know little about its use. Most physicians in hospitals have heard of the possible use of acupuncture instead of anesthesia, but it is also becoming more accepted in other areas, such as minimizing pain and nausea for the patient once the operation is over and the patient is in the recovery room. Acupuncture also has some interesting uses possible in emergency room treatments.

The AAMA is also very dedicated to pursuing research and studies into new applications for acupuncture in both the hospital and physician office settings. It is especially interested in researchers to look into the fundamentals of why certain acupuncture techniques are as successful as they are. In other words, many doctors want a traditional medical explanation of the process that the acupuncture treatment starts. It seems that a simple insertion of a number of needles is a mystifying way to accomplish the results, and there is a good deal of research into how to exactly explain the mechanisms that occur. Doctors who do research into these areas may publish their results in a magazine called

Medical Acupuncture is the official journal of the American Academy of Medical Acupuncture. The magazine presents authoritative papers, case reports, and research findings that integrate concepts from traditional and modern forms of acupuncture with Western medical training. This publication covers the effectiveness and safety of acupuncture in pain relief, cancer, stroke, pulmonology, urology, OB/GYN, gastroenterology, and much more.

The existence of a large and growing numbers of qualified physicians that are also trained acupuncturists' guarantees that the benefits of each discipline will continue to make current American health practice better for the patients.

How to Find an Acupuncture Practitioner

Finding an acupuncture practitioner is much easier now that it is a much more common means of therapy. You can find one the same way you find a dentist, by simply looking on the internet, in the phone book, or asking one of your friends that is knowledgeable about current health advances. There are several national acupuncture organizations on the Internet, and you can look up your locality by state and city. You can also ask your family physician, for more and more doctors are referring their patients to an acupuncture clinic for the treatment of certain problems. You might be even more surprised to find that your doctor or internist may have training in acupuncture themselves, or one of the associated therapies.

Once you find several acupuncture practitioners in your area, you should make sure to check their credentials. This is always a good idea for you to do for all of your health support team, from your internist to your dentist. Not all states have established training standards required for acupuncture certification, but if yours does, ask the acupuncture practitioner about their training, background, and certifications. Although a certification does not ensure an excellent practitioner, you are at least assured that they have had sufficient training in the area. Do not rely on your practitioner to diagnose a disease unless they have conventional medical training. An acupuncturist is well trained to observe and address symptoms, but the Chinese medicine behind acupuncture is not particularly concerned about naming a specific disease. If you have significant symptoms that you feel needs a precise diagnosis, rely on a trained doctor. As mentioned earlier, your doctor may encourage you to seek the services of an acupuncture clinic to address certain symptoms that you may have.

Once you have found out the background of the acupuncture practitioners, the decision to select one is similar to the decision that you use to select a dentist. You may have friends that recommend them, you may schedule an initial visit and see how you feel at the office, etc. The remainder of the decision is more on how comfortable you feel with that acupuncture practitioner. The initial visit will consist of a diagnosis, where you will talk at length with the practitioner, and that will give you a very good indication of whether you are comfortable or not.

The cost of the treatments will be discussed after your diagnosis. The number of treatments will depend on your set of symptoms and your overall health. The acupuncture practitioner should discuss this before the series of treatments start. Some symptoms only require a few treatments, whereas others may stretch over a series of weeks. Typically, physicians that are also trained in acupuncture will charge more than nonphysicians.

Your insurance may cover visits to the acupuncture clinic, but you should contact them first and discuss your individual case. Make sure to mention whether it is a referral from your physician, if indeed it is. This introduction has hopefully given you the information you need to confidently find and schedule your first acupuncture clinic visit!

Most physicians who practice acupuncture, regardless of their specialty, are likely to be of assistance regarding your symptom. We suggest you find an AAMA member near you and call their office. If they do not treat patients with your condition their office is still a wonderful resource for a referral to someone they would recommend in your area.

www.ingramcontent.com/pod-product-compliance
Lightning Source LLC
Chambersburg PA
CBHW071624170526
45166CB00003B/1184